WEIGHT LO
DIET BOOK
FOR OBESE
CHILDREN

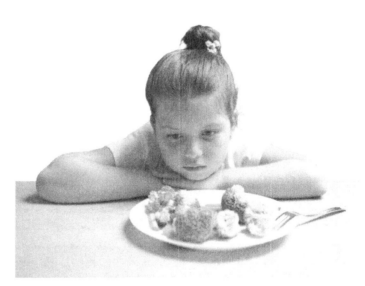

A guide on how to prevent
and reduce obesity in children
and adolescents

Sharon J. Beeman

TABLE OF CONTENTS

INTRODUCTION

Lynn's son was a happy and active child, but he was also overweight. He was constantly teased by his peers and struggled to keep up with them during physical activities. Lynn was worried about her son's health and decided to take action. She consulted with a nutritionist and developed a weight loss diet specifically tailored to her son's needs.

The diet was designed to help him lose weight in a healthy and sustainable way, while still providing him with the nutrition he needed to grow and develop. Through this diet, Lynn's son was able to lose weight and become more active and confident. He was able to enjoy physical activities with his peers and was no longer the target of teasing. Lynn's story is a testament to the power of a healthy diet in helping children achieve their weight loss goals.

Obesity in children is fast becoming an issue of concern in the United States. It can lead to a variety of health issues, including heart disease, diabetes, and high blood pressure. To help combat this problem, parents must take an active role in their children's health and nutrition.

One way to do this is to create a weight loss diet specifically tailored to their child's needs. This diet should be designed to help the child lose weight in a healthy and sustainable way, while still providing them with the nutrition they need to grow and develop. Lynn's story is a great example of how a weight loss diet can help an obese child achieve their goals.

With the help of the tips in this book you will learn how to create a weight loss diet for your child that is tailored to their individual needs. You will learn how to make healthy food choices, how to create a balanced meal plan, and how to motivate your child to stick to their diet. By following these tips, you can help your child achieve their weight loss goals and lead a healthier life.

CHAPTER 1
NUTRITION BASICS.

1.Eating healthy: Eating healthy is very important in weight loss. Consuming a variety of foods from each dietary group, such as fruits, vegetables, whole grains, lean proteins, and healthy fats, is necessary to achieve this.

2. Reduce your intake of processed foods: These foods tend to be heavy in calories, fat, sugar, and sodium, which can lead to weight gain. Aim to consume fewer processed foods and more freshly prepared, complete foods.

3. Increase your intake of fibre: Fibre helps you feel fuller for longer and might lessen cravings. With whole grains, fruits, vegetables, and legumes, try to consume at least 25 to 30 grams of fibre per day.

4 Sip lots of water. Water helps you stay hydrated and might help you feel less hungry. The target is to drink at least 8 glasses of water each day.

5. Limit added sugars: Added sugars can cause weight gain and are included in many processed foods. Limit added sugars and choose natural sweeteners as much as possible.

6. Get enough sleep: Sleep is crucial for shedding pounds. Ensure that you take adequate rest of not less than 8 hours each night.

7. Get moving: Exercise is essential for shedding pounds and maintaining good health. Aim for 60 minutes or more of physical activity each day.

8. Keep an eye on portion sizes: Portion sizes can significantly affect weight loss. Try to keep an eye on your portion sizes and choose lesser servings whenever you can.

9. Consume food slowly. Eating slowly can assist prevent overeating and encourage weight loss. Just eat to enjoy your food by savouring every bite.

10. Prevent skipping meals: Skipping meals might result in binge eating later in the day, which can hinder weight loss. Try to eat regular meals all day long.

CHAPTER 2
MACRONUTRIENTS

Macronutrients are the three main components of food that provide energy and nutrition to the body: carbohydrates, proteins, and fats. They are essential for growth and development, and for maintaining a healthy weight.

In obese children, macronutrients play an important role in helping to reduce excess body fat and improve overall health. Carbohydrates are the body's main source of energy and should make up the majority of a child's diet.

Complex carbohydrates, such as whole grains, fruits, and vegetables, are the best sources of carbohydrates.

These foods are high in fibre, which helps to keep the digestive system healthy and can help to reduce hunger. Eating a variety of complex carbohydrates can also help to provide essential vitamins and minerals.

Proteins are important for growth and development, and for maintaining muscle mass. Lean proteins, such as fish, poultry, and beans, are the best sources of protein. Eating lean proteins can help to reduce hunger and provide essential amino acids.

Fats are an important part of a healthy diet, but it is important to choose healthy fats. Unsaturated fats, such as those found in nuts, seeds, and avocados, are the best sources of fat. Eating healthy fats can help to reduce hunger and provide essential fatty acids.

Obese children should focus on eating a balanced diet that includes all three macronutrients. Eating a variety of complex carbohydrates, lean proteins, and healthy fats can help to reduce excess body fat and improve overall health. It is also important to limit processed and sugary foods, as these can contribute to weight gain. Eating a balanced diet and getting regular physical activity can help to reduce the risk of obesity and improve overall health.

MICRONUTRIENTS

Micronutrients are essential vitamins and minerals that are required in small amounts for the body to function properly. Micronutrients are present basically in fruits, vegetables, grains, and dairy products. In children, micronutrients are especially important for growth and development.

Obese children are at risk for a variety of health problems, including diabetes, heart disease, and other chronic conditions. In addition, they may be deficient in certain micronutrients due to their poor dietary habits. A lack of micronutrients can lead to a variety of health problems, including anaemia, weakened bones, and impaired cognitive development.

It is important for obese children to get adequate amounts of micronutrients in their diets. Their diet or meal plan should be made to include varieties of fruits, vegetables, whole grains, and lean proteins that can help ensure that the required micronutrients they need are gotten. Additionally, obese children should be encouraged to engage in regular physical activity, as this can help them burn calories and improve their overall health.

In addition to dietary changes, obese children may benefit from taking a multivitamin or other supplement to ensure that they are getting all of the micronutrients they need. However, it is important to consult with a doctor or nutritionist before starting any supplement regimen.

Overall, micronutrients are essential for the health and development of all children, including those who are obese. Eating a balanced diet and engaging in regular physical activity can help ensure that obese children get the micronutrients they need. Additionally, a doctor or nutritionist may recommend a multivitamin or other supplement to help ensure that they are getting all of the micronutrients they need.

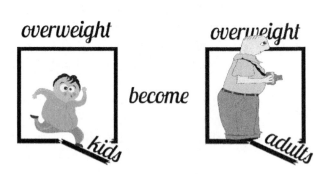

CHAPTER 3
MEAL PLANNING

When planning a meal for an obese child the following should be taken into consideration.

1. **Choose nutrient-dense foods:** Focus on providing meals that are high in vitamins, minerals, and fibre, and low in calories, saturated fat, and added sugars.

2. **Limit processed foods:** Avoid processed foods that are high in calories, fat, and sugar.

3. **Include plenty of fruits and vegetables:** Fruits and vegetables are packed with vitamins, minerals, and fibre, and are low in calories.

4. **Include lean proteins:** Lean proteins such as fish, poultry, and beans are a great source of protein and can help keep your child full and satisfied.

5. **Limit added sugars:** Added sugars can add extra calories to meals without providing any nutritional value.

6. **Encourage physical activity**: Regular physical activity can help your child maintain a healthy weight.

7. **Monitor portion sizes:** Make sure your child is eating appropriate portion sizes for their age and activity level.

8. **Avoid skipping meals:** Skipping meals can lead to overeating later in the day.

Here is an example of an ideal meal plan.

Breakfast

-Whole wheat toast with peanut butter
-1 cup of low-fat milk
-1 piece of fresh fruit

Lunch

-Turkey sandwich on whole wheat bread
-1 cup of vegetable soup

-1 cup of low-fat yoghurts
Snack
-1 cup of air-popped popcorn
-1 piece of fresh fruit
Dinner
-Grilled chicken breast
-1 cup of steamed vegetables
-1/2 cup of cooked brown rice
Dessert
-1/2 cup of low-fat frozen yoghourt
-1/4 cup of fresh berries

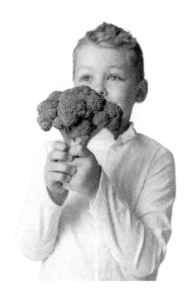

CHAPTER 4
EXERCISE

Exercises should be encouraged for an obese child. Exercise can help an obese child to burn calories, build muscle, and improve overall health. The most important thing is to start slowly and increase the intensity and duration of the exercise gradually and also more importantly ensure the child is having fun while exercising.

A 60 minutes moderate to vigorous physical activity should be encouraged for children and adolescents between the ages of 6 to 17 as recommended by the American Academy of Pediatrics. These exercises include aerobics, muscle-strengthening exercises and also bone-strengthening exercises.This should guide your weight loss plan.

Cardio

For an obese child, it is important to focus on low-impact cardio exercises that are safe and effective. Examples of such exercises include walking, swimming, biking, and jogging. Additionally, activities such as hula hooping, jump roping, and dancing can be great ways to get the heart rate up and burn calories.

It is important to ensure that the child is comfortable with the activity and that it is done in a safe environment.

Strength Training

Strength training for an obese child should be approached with caution. It is important to consult with a doctor or physical therapist before beginning any type of strength training program. Generally, strength training for an obese child should focus on low-impact exercises that are designed to

improve overall strength and endurance.
Examples of low-impact exercises include bodyweight exercises such as squats, lunges, and push-ups, as well as light weightlifting with dumbbells or resistance bands. It is important to ensure that the child is using proper form and technique to avoid injury. Additionally, it is important to ensure that the child is not overtraining and is taking adequate rest days.

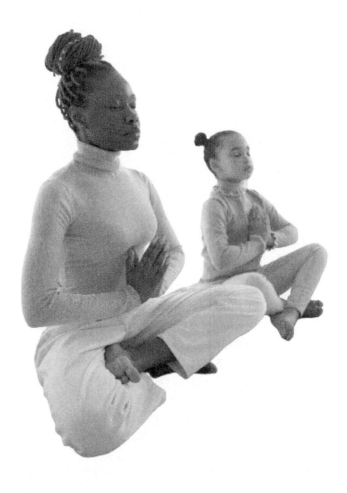

CHAPTER 5
DIET RECIPES AND
SMOOTHIES .

Day 1
Breakfast

Overnight oats with banana and almond milk (10 minutes prep time)

Lunch

Grilled chicken and vegetable wrap (15 minutes prep time)

Snack

Apple slices with peanut butter (5 minutes prep time)

Dinner

Baked salmon with roasted vegetables (20 minutes prep time)

Day 2
Breakfast

Scrambled eggs with spinach and mushrooms (10 minutes prep time)

Lunch

Turkey and cheese sandwich on whole wheat bread (10 minutes prep time)

Snack

Celery sticks with hummus (5 minutes prep time)

Dinner

Baked chicken with quinoa and steamed broccoli (20 minutes prep time)

Day 3
Breakfast

Greek yoghourt with berries and granola (10 minutes prep time)

Lunch

Tuna salad wrap (10 minutes prep time)

Snack

Carrot sticks with guacamole (5 minutes prep time)

Dinner

Baked cod with roasted sweet potatoes and asparagus (20 minutes prep time)

Day 4
Breakfast

Oatmeal with banana and walnuts (10 minutes prep time)

Lunch

Turkey and avocado sandwich on whole wheat bread (10 minutes prep time)

Snack

Apple slices with almond butter (5 minutes prep time)

Dinner

Baked salmon with quinoa and steamed vegetables (20 minutes prep time)

Day 5
Breakfast

Smoothie bowl with banana, berries, and almond milk (10 minutes prep time)

Lunch

Grilled chicken and vegetable wrap (15 minutes prep time)

Snack

Celery sticks with peanut butter (5 minutes prep time)

Dinner

Baked cod with roasted potatoes and green beans (20 minutes prep time)

Day 6
Breakfast

Scrambled eggs with spinach and tomatoes (10 minutes prep time)

Lunch

Hummus and vegetable wrap (10 minutes prep time)

Snack

Carrot sticks with hummus (5 minutes prep time)

Dinner

Baked chicken with quinoa and steamed broccoli (20 minutes prep time)

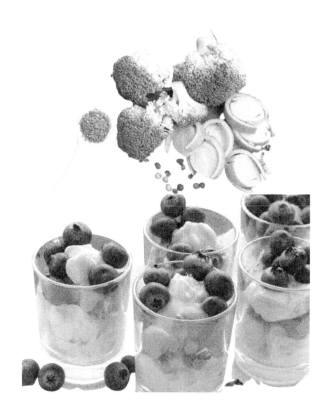

Day 7

Breakfast

Overnight oats with banana and almond milk (10 minutes prep time)

Lunch

Turkey and cheese sandwich on whole wheat bread (10 minutes prep time)

Snack

Apple slices with almond butter (5 minutes prep time)

Dinner

Baked salmon with roasted vegetables (20 minutes prep time).

5 SMOOTHIES RECIPES YOUR CHILD WILL ENJOY

Banana-Mango Smoothie
Blend 1 banana, 1 cup of frozen mango chunks, 1/2 cup of plain Greek yoghurt, 1/2 cup of orange juice, and 1/4 teaspoon of ground cinnamon until smooth.

Strawberry-Kiwi Smoothie
Blend 1 cup of frozen strawberries, 1 kiwi, peeled and sliced, 1/2 cup of plain Greek yoghurt, 1/4 cup of almond milk, and 1/4 teaspoon of ground ginger until smooth.

Blueberry-Coconut Smoothie
Blend 1 cup of frozen blueberries, 1/2 cup of plain Greek yoghurt, 1/4 cup of coconut milk, 1/4 teaspoon of ground cardamom, and 1 tablespoon of honey until smooth.

Peach-Almond Smoothie
 Blend 1 cup of frozen peaches, 1/2 cup of plain Greek yoghurt, 1/4 cup of almond milk, 1/4 teaspoon of ground cinnamon, and 1 tablespoon of honey until smooth.

Pineapple-Coconut Smoothie
 Blend 1 cup of frozen pineapple chunks, 1/2 cup of plain Greek yoghurt, 1/4 cup of coconut milk, 1/4 teaspoon of ground nutmeg, and 1 tablespoon of honey until smooth.

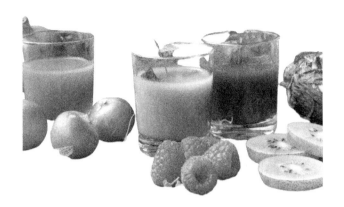

CONCLUSION

In conclusion, a weight loss diet for obese children should be tailored to the individual child's needs and preferences. Be sure to include nutrient-dense foods, such as fruits, vegetables, whole grains, lean proteins, and also healthy fats. It should also include regular physical activity and lifestyle changes to help promote healthy weight loss. Parents should work with their child's healthcare provider to ensure that the diet is safe and effective.

With the right diet and lifestyle changes, obese children can achieve a healthy weight and reduce their risk of developing chronic diseases. Obese kids may feel embarrassed, ashamed, and isolated. They may also feel judged and discriminated against by their peers and adults. They may feel like they don't fit in and struggle with low self-esteem.

They may also feel overwhelmed and frustrated by the physical and emotional challenges of being overweight. As a parent you can help your child by encouraging healthy habits such as eating right and healthy regular exercise and getting adequate rest.

Commend their efforts as this will help them to focus on the process rather than the outcome.

Model healthy behaviour for your child by eating healthy foods, exercising regularly, and maintaining a positive attitude. Spend time with your child especially in doing activities that they enjoy making them feel loved. Talk to your child about body image and how it is not related to their worth and also encourage your child to talk positively about themselves and their body and most importantly by sticking to the tips in this book you will be able to create a healthy weight loss diet for your child that will help them reach their goals and build a healthier lifestyle and boost their confidence and self-esteem.

Printed in Great Britain
by Amazon

43380634R00020